
STOMACH VACUUMS
EXPLAINED

JAMES DRIVER

Contents

Introduction

The stomach vacuum has been used for thousands of years. Although it's not known precisely when or where the technique was first practised, or by whom, what is known is that it's been used by Shaolin monks at their famed temple in Henan Province, China, for centuries.

Across the Asian continent in India, a version of the stomach vacuum, Udiyan Bandh, also known as the abdominal lock or upward lifting lock, has been used for at least the last thousand years, though probably a lot longer.

More recently, the stomach vacuum was extremely popular during the golden age of bodybuilding, from the 1950s to the 1970s, including by such champions as Arnold Schwarzenegger. Compare side by side the abdomen of Arnold in his prime to your everyday modern bodybuilder and notice the difference between the Austrian Oak's concave, inward curving belly and the more flattened, even convex outward curving shape of his modern-day counterparts, despite them often possessing very visible abdominals (the coveted six-pack), including a prominent line down the middle (linea alba).

It's quite easy to tell which of your favourite social media fitness people perform stomach vacuums and those who don't as there's a subtle yet marked difference in the curvature of their abdomens, something that's becoming increasingly easier to spot the more of a trained eye you develop.

Why the difference in aesthetic? In Arnold's own words, it's because "These days, it seems almost nobody does the vacuum anymore. I suppose that with the increased bodyweights of competitors come bigger midsections and, as a result, less ability to suck up into a vacuum. There is such an overemphasis on getting heavy that too little attention is paid to controlling the growth of the waistline."

It appears that all of a sudden, and for no good reason in particular, narrower waistlines were no longer desired as the world forgot all about the stomach vacuum.

Which brings me to the reason for writing what will be a relatively short book covering this one simple, yet very effective exercise technique for achieving a slimmer waist, among other benefits that you'll soon discover.

I also have another reason for writing this book. As a fitness enthusiast, keen weightlifter, HIIT fanatic as well as the best-selling author of HIIT: High Intensity Interval Training Explained, and a university lecturer on the subject of Sport Science, it irked me greatly to read some of the misleading online content with regards the stomach vacuum. This content ranged from improper instructions of how to perform the exercise to both deflated and immensely inflated claims about its effectiveness and potency, such as;

"This practice is considered to be one of the easiest ways to burn fat!"

"Feel the fat melt away with the stomach vacuum!"

"This is the single best way of achieving your dream ab-look."

Perhaps most remarkable of all, one popular fitness site published an article confusing stomach vacuums, the exercise, with stomach vacuum therapy, despite them being two completely different things, and cited the results of a study into the latter as the reason why you should be doing the former.

With all this internet noise, I felt it was time to come out of book retirement and write another, albeit, short book, if only to set the record straight and provide a simple and realistic explanation of the stomach vacuum, its benefits (there are many and they are great), its limitations as well as drawbacks, how to properly perform it and how to progress with it.

So, with all that said, let's begin with an explanation of the large and very important muscle the stomach vacuum targets.

The Transverse Abdominis - The Body's Corset Muscle

The transverse abdominis (TA) is a large, band-like muscle located deep, or below, the internal obliques and rectus abdominis, or six-pack. Where the abdominals run vertically, the TA is a horizontal muscle that reaches around the midsection like a corset, protecting the spine and quite literally holding in your guts.

Vertically, at the anterior, the TA arises from several origins, one of which is the lower six ribs, it then interlocks with the diaphragm and inserts into the pubis. Horizontally, the TA inserts into the linea alba, the vertical line separating the abdominals.

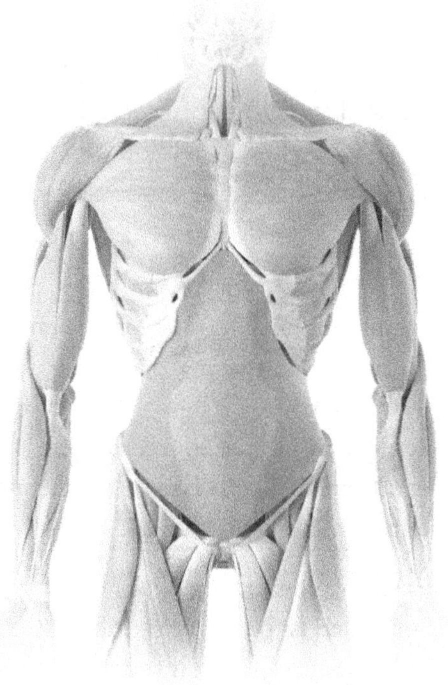

The transverse abdominis is the deepest of the core muscles.

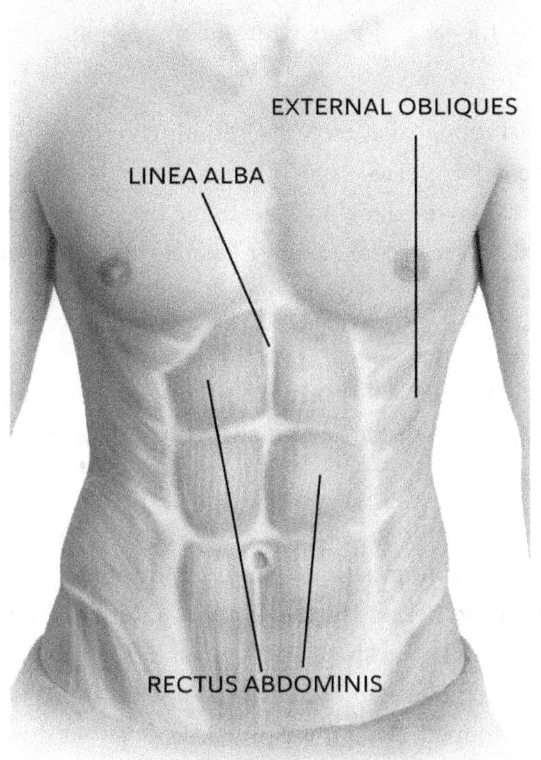

The muscles of the abdomen.

The TA is crucial for the health of your core and back, its primary purpose being to compress the ribs and contents of the abdomen for stability, the muscle fibres indeed acting like a large belt, effectively pulling everything together and preventing the abdomen from protruding outwards. When walking into a roomful of people, it's the TA you can thank for, either consciously or unconsciously, reducing the size of your belly when you pull everything in.

Whilst training the rectus abdominis with a series of crunches, leg raises and dragon flags will eventually bestow the coveted six-pack aesthetic upon the participant, body fat levels excepted, these exercises alone will not in any way serve to flatten the belly beyond which they employ the TA secondarily.

For women, the TA also supports babies during pregnancy, and together with the uterus and pelvic floor muscles, it's this muscle that works to push the baby out during delivery.

Whilst performing a great range of lifts the TA contracts involuntarily, acting as the body's natural weightlifting belt to stabilize the spine and pelvis. Being the deepest of the core muscles, lifting heavy weights with an underdeveloped TA is the equivalent of attempting to fire a cannon from a small boat; it might be easy enough with a 6-pounder firing off the port side but as soon as you bring out the 32 then you're liable to have difficulties. Let me be clear, you might still be able to lift the heavy weight, as the cannon might even be able to deliver its payload without tearing off half the hull in a cloud of splinters, but by first building a solid core foundation you're sure to find making those heavier lifts far easier, which will then, in turn, aid further progression.

Typically, an untrained muscle will remain in its lengthened state. An untrained upper back will result in a posture where the shoulders round forwards, particularly if the chest is indeed trained and developed out of unison with its opposing muscles. Another example is the quadriceps, which are often overtrained when compared to their antagonist, the hamstrings. This muscle imbalance is what leads to a great many knee problems, not to mention hindrance when it comes to progression with a range of other lifts. When a muscle contracts it shortens - The TA can be trained in the same way as any other muscle and by doing so it will act, shortening that corset, and pulling in the abdomen of its own accord and without any conscious effort on the part of the individual, even at rest. Aesthetically, and again because untrained muscles remain in their lengthened states, a lack of training in this area might well result in a distended, protruding lower abdomen.

Even without an excess of belly fat the abdomen can still stick out. Indeed, even with a well-trained rectus abdominis coupled with exceptionally low levels of body fat, it's still possible to suffer from belly protrusion, especially if the participant has never, or has seldom, targeted the TA specifically.

Of course, factors like poor posture, bloating and genetics can also make your belly project outwards, though genetics should never be used as an excuse when the fix is as simple as dedicating a few minutes a day towards targeting the TA with a series of stomach vacuums. Recall Arnie's quote from above, "These days, it seems almost nobody does the vacuum anymore." Let's compare side by side Arnold Schwarzenegger in his prime to a modern contemporary.

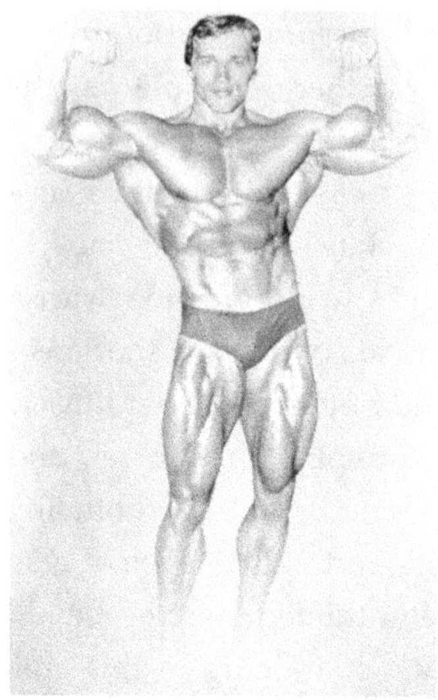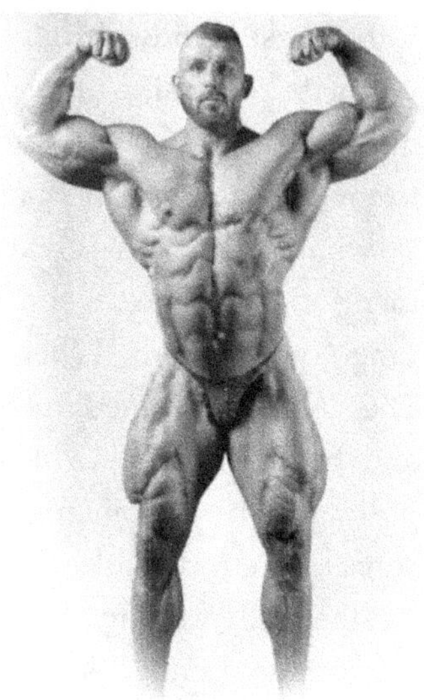

As you can see, Arnold possesses a concave, inward curving abdomen that further visually enhances his wide lats and shoulders. Andrea Muzi, on the other hand, has quite a convex, outward curving stomach that serves to detract from the wide aesthetic he'd otherwise own. This despite having a far more prominent six-pack than Arnold.

Of course, these two gentlemen are extreme examples, and there are many far more prominent cases of these convex shapes if you care to look (my use of images was limited for reasons of copyright), but I hope I've made the point that you can indeed be totally ripped and still suffer from a protruding abdomen, in which case there is a far greater likelihood that we mere mortals, those of us who're not professional bodybuilders and who just desire a flatter abdomen, might also be experiencing a similar disposition.

Fortunately, there is a solution, and that solution is the simple employment of a long neglected exercise.

2

Vacuums, Maneuvers, Exercises - It's All So Confusing

I think that at this point it might be useful to clear up any confusion with regards to stomach vacuums and some of the other exercises or treatments that may be similar in nature, or in the case of the first one, almost the same in name and yet completely different in reality.

Stomach Vacuum Therapy

I would have preferred not to mention vacuum therapy in this book at all, but for the names being so similar, and the before mentioned confusion having already occurred, I thought it best to clear up any more conflation that might potentially follow.

Not to be confused with stomach vacuums, the subject of this book, stomach or abdominal vacuum therapy, or vacuum cupping therapy, on the other hand, is something completely different.

Whereas stomach vacuums are exercises you actively carry out, vacuum therapy is a 'body contouring' procedure that's done passively to you, often by a therapist whilst lying back on a table. Neither is vacuum therapy a procedure that's carried out merely to your stomach, but the thighs, arms, back and bum can also be targeted.

If you follow certain fitness enthusiasts on social media then you might well have seen images of suction cups attached to a mechanical device that massages the flesh, and then the large red circles left behind afterwards, indeed, it's owing to the fresh exposure from celebrities that's given this ancient technique a fresh boost. The beneficial claims made by practitioners include; improved digestion, relaxation (it feels like being massaged) and a way of relieving pain and fatigue, as well as aiding recovery. While it's claimed by some that applying suction cups to the abdomen and other areas will help target fat for faster metabolization, the likelihood is that this technique does little beyond that of a massage, helping you to better recover before the next training session and can therefore be considered a tertiary aid at best.

Ignore claims made by proponents of cupping such as "drains belly fat fast."

To further confuse matters we can also add vacuum RF (Radio Frequency) therapy. Although marketed more as a skin exfoliating measure and cellulite treatment rather than a way of reducing fat or waist circumference, confusion still exists. This procedure involves applying oil before running a paddle combining radio frequency, lasers, suction and massage to the target area. Though little scientific literature on this treatment exists, the American Board of Cosmetic Surgery has suggested that any positive effects are minimal and temporary at best.

A search for any one of stomach vacuums, stomach vacuum therapy or stomach vacuum RF therapy will yield results for all three, and it's this which has caused much confusion, even within articles published in prominent journals, magazines and websites.

Abdominal Draw-in Manoeuvre

Like the Fartlek method is to the HIIT or Tabata workout, the abdominal draw-in manoeuvre is an easier version of the stomach vacuum. Where with the stomach vacuum the idea is to go 'all-out' with a strong and intense contraction and then spending a short while recovering before the next repetition (more on this soon), the abdominal draw-in manoeuvre entails shorter repetitions, frequent stops for breath, and less intense contractions. For those participants wishing to begin stomach vacuums by dipping their feet into something easier, I will be providing details on progression later. Whether you wish to call repetitions at the less intense side of the spectrum *easy stomach vacuums* or *abdominal draw-ins* is up to you.

Stomach/Abdominal Hollowing

Again, this can be thought of as a less intense version of the stomach vacuum, with repetitions lasting for as short a time as two seconds. Additionally, abdominal exercises involving the legs, such as wipers, flutter kicks or scissor manoeuvres are often incorporated. Whilst adding an extra dimension, and no doubt making a fine workout for the core muscles, my feeling is that the TA muscle, although definitely activated, does not receive the isolation and concentration it deserves and would otherwise get with full-on stomach vacuums.

With all that out of the way, let's now move on to learn more about the subject of this book.

3

Stomach Vacuums - History's Most Under Appreciated Exercise?

Stomach vacuums are a well-known exercise from the 1970s when many trainers began noticing the effect they had on the waistlines and abdomens of bodybuilders. Though as already stated, it's not merely bodybuilders from the Golden Age who're familiar with this exercise. In yoga, the stomach vacuum is named Udiyan Bandh, or the abdominal lock, and is often performed during workouts. Other than that, I wish I could cite more examples but as you can see, the stomach vacuum happens to be one of the most neglected techniques by both professional athletes and recreational exercisers alike.

The stomach vacuum is an isometric exercise, which means that the muscle, in this case the TA, is contracting without moving. Other examples of isometric exercises would include standing side-on to a wall, arms against your sides, whilst pressing the back of your hand as hard as you can against it in order to contract the deltoids. You could also stack a weights machine with so many plates that there's no hope of moving it. Why do this? Because the longer your muscles struggle against a given load the more muscle fibres are recruited to complete the task. It's for this reason that when compared to either concentric or eccentric contractions (the up and down movements respectively), isometric contractions yield superior strength increases [1,2,3,4] whilst reducing fatigue [1]. The disadvantage, however, is that this superior strength increase occurs only within that small degree of motion where the isometric contraction is held [1]. As it happens, this is excellent news and no disadvantage at all when considering the stomach vacuum, for the obvious reason that when it comes to the TA there's only that small degree of motion where we really want and require that strength increase to occur, which is as cinched in as we can realistically make it, and this is the spot you'll be aiming to hold your contractions.

As already discussed, vacuums target the TA but also to a lesser extent both the internal and external obliques. As expected, however, activation of the six-pack during this exercise has been shown to be very low [5].

Benefits of Stomach Vacuums

Let's now take a look at some of the various benefits that come from performing this exercise.

Increased postural support and stability

It's known that the spinal stabilizer muscles, pelvic floor muscles and the muscles of the deep trunk, which includes the TA, play a major role in postural stability. A review of the existing literature [6] suggests that physical training that focuses on this region improves postural control.

A study involving 24 female college-age dancers [7] performed the abdominal draw-in manoeuvre three times a week for nine weeks, after which significant improvements were found in single-leg balance, both static and dynamic, and the ability to pirouette.

Using a broader sample of non-athletes [8], 125 females aged 18-60 were randomly selected to either an experimental group carrying out two sessions per week of stomach vacuums lasting 30 minutes, or a control group who did not receive the treatment, after which balance and postural control were assessed by the use of a stabilometric platform. At the conclusion of the study, the group engaging in stomach vacuums were found to have significantly improved postural stability.

Helps with lifts and injury prevention

Remember that the TA is our body's version of a weight belt. Frequent intentional contraction of this belt helps us to gain control over the entire core, thus protecting against injury by increasing intra-abdominal pressure and bracing the spine. This also provides assistance with a great many lifts, particularly the heavy compound lifts performed when standing, such as the deadlift, squat, standing military press, as well as the more explosive lifts like cleans, jerks and snatches.

Pain relief

A common occurrence when it comes to back pain is going about your daily routine without a TA that contracts when needed. This can encompass all tasks from sitting up in a chair or getting out of bed to carrying heavy objects or bracing against a fall, if your TA is not contracting to keep everything nice and compact then pain can easily result.

A study [9] involving women with lower back pain aged 40-49 found that using the abdominal draw-in manoeuvre resulted in decreased pain and reduced dysfunctions in the lumbar region. Of course, this study used the less intense version of the stomach vacuum, which is an unfortunate limitation when it comes to the subject of this book, but I have no reason to doubt that results would only continue to improve for these subjects if, in their own time, they progressed to what I'm advocating for here.

A treatment for diastasis recti abdominis

Diastasis recti abdominis (DRA) refers to the separation of the abdominal muscles, specifically a widening of the linea alba, the midline that runs down the centre. DRA most commonly occurs after pregnancy, having been found [10] to affect up to 60% of women either during pregnancy or postpartum, although some studies [11] suggest that when it comes to non-exercising women the number might be as high as 90%. DRA can also occur as a result of lifting heavy weights or unsafe abdominal exercise practices. This condition is capable of allowing a bulge or "pooch" to form in the abdomen, in fact, this *is* the most common reported symptom of DRA. Lower back pain, bloating, constipation and poor posture may also manifest as symptoms, as well as the consequent hindrance when it comes to performing daily tasks, and can last for months, if not many years.

It should not be surprising, therefore, that decreasing the severity of DRA separation can be extremely beneficial to a sufferer's daily living conditions as well as psychological wellbeing.

The importance of contracting the TA, in particular, has been noted for bringing together the bellies of the rectus abdominis, ameliorating abdominal protrusion, improving the integrity of the linea alba and thereby reducing DRA [12], and which may also positively impact postpartum body satisfaction [13].

In 2014, a paper [14] reviewing the existing literature on the phenomenon (eight studies totalling 300+ postnatal females) found that exercise reduced the presence of DRA by 35%. Unfortunately, and owing to the existing literature being of poor quality, the paper did not specify which exercises were undertaken. This, I have found whilst researching this book, has been a problem for me too, as studies concerning the TA, and stomach vacuums in particular, are sadly lacking. However, with regards DRA I was to strike lucky, as a new paper [12] examining the effectiveness of an online 12-week exercise intervention on the condition within a sample of postpartum women became available just as I was at the planning stages (and deciding whether or not I should continue).

Eight postpartum women took part in the study, measuring the width of the linea alba at baseline and 12 weeks post-intervention, at three different locations; the navel and both two inches above and below the navel at both rest and during the stomach vacuums for a total of six readings. The study concluded with findings that after 12 weeks of stomach vacuums, there were moderate decreases in linea alba width both above and below the navel, both at rest and during the exercise activity.

These findings are extremely positive, though one might be tempted to be sceptical, postulating that perhaps several of these mothers had only just given birth and that therefore 12 weeks is sufficient enough time for the abdominal muscles to heal naturally. As it happens, the study subjects possessed a 14-month postpartum mean, which is easily long enough for the extent of any natural healing that was to take place to have already happened.

On their own, stomach vacuums can provide meaningful improvements for treating DRA, but of course they should encompass only a portion of a young mother's exercise regimen.

Fights protrusion of the stomach

I'm under no illusion that this is the single greatest reason why most people are reading these words. I don't want to make any bold claims with regards exactly how much stomach vacuums could decrease the size of your waistline because I think this is one of those things that has many factors to it, not least existing body fat percentages, but also somatotype (body shape), gender, child-birthing as well as the possibility of diastasis recti abdominis, bloating, other medical conditions, race (body fat can be stored in different quantities depending on the location), as well as past exercise activity, particularly with regards to abdominal exercises, which altogether means that results will almost certainly be different for every participant.

What we can be sure about are the following fundamentals:

- The transverse abdominis holds your internal organs in place, preventing them from protruding outwards
- By contracting the transverse abdominis, your internal organs will compress
- The stomach vacuum exercise is by far the best way of contracting the transverse abdominis
- An exercised/trained muscle will remain in a relatively more contracted state as opposed to an untrained muscle, which will be more inclined to remain elongated

With this said we can reasonably postulate:

- That newly added strength will assist with pulling in your internal organs and giving you a slimmer waistline as well as more abdominal control. Over time you may see a significant difference in the flatness of your stomach.

It's to this end that perhaps it's only logical that instructional video and article comment sections regarding this topic are crammed with personal anecdotes of "I lost 2 inches,' or "I lost 3 inches in only a few weeks."

Although there are many, many anecdotes of stomach vacuums helping individuals tighten their midsections and reduce the circumference of their waists, sometimes by significant margins, astonishingly there are very few, if any, peer-reviewed studies with the specific intention of discovering if it's the stomach vacuum specifically, rather than a combination of other lifestyle related factors (dieting and other exercises), that can be attributed to the reductions. Unfortunately, most, if not all the studies, appear to measure waist circumference only as a secondary component, almost as an afterthought, to the original study aims.

Take for example this study [15] conducted in Spain in 2016. Stomach vacuums, which they called the hypopressive technique, were used on 11 female Rugby players in order to assess changes in pelvic floor function. Measurements of body composition were made and naturally, because waist to hip ratio is one of the classic methods of recording this metric, data on waist circumference was attained. I'm sure you're curious - the results showed that stomach vacuums do indeed increase the maximum contractility and muscle tone of the pelvic floor muscles, so it looks like the exercise that is the subject of this book can now also add bladder control to its list of attributes. As for the afterthought - not surprisingly, no change in hip circumference was noted, for *waist* circumference, however, after 8 weeks of performing 45-

minute sessions of stomach vacuums twice per week, the mean average reduction at this location was 2.68 cm (1.06 inches), significantly greater than the control group.

This may or may not sound like a lot to you, depending on what your goals are, though it's important to remember that eight weeks is not a great deal of time outside of a study setting, and that also this study was conducted on Rugby players, women who were already athletes and whom undoubtedly already undergo strict physical regimens that in some cases might already have included some form of stomach vacuum component. For the average individual, however, particularly those who're merely wishing to get back into shape and improve upon their physical appearance then stomach vacuums should only ever encompass a portion of their overall fitness plan regardless, which brings us to the next section.

Stomach vacuums do not burn fat

I've been left astonished by some of the misleading claims regarding stomach vacuums, often within reputable publications, and it was some of these claims that prompted me to write this book. Let me make this clear:

Stomach vacuums do not burn fat!

They very well may help reduce your waistline, and therefore should be used as a supplementary exercise, but we should never lose sight of the fact that the bread and butter of weight/fat loss and/or waist reduction should always be:

- A moderately aggressive reduction in calories to a level below your daily caloric requirements.
- An increase in protein intake at the expense of carbohydrates. A suggested macronutrient ratio is 40/40/20 (carbs/protein/fat) to progress to 35/40/25 (carbs/protein/fat) when hitting a plateau.
- A weightlifting regimen to signal to your body that muscle mass should be retained at the expense of body fat.
- A HIIT workout twice per week, to be increased to three times per week when hitting a plateau. When it comes to fat loss, HIIT has been shown to be nine times more efficient than steady-state cardio [16].
- Supplementary light cardio work such as walking can be added later, and is best added incrementally to break plateaus.

That's it! The longer you remain in this state then the more fat you will burn and by incorporating stomach vacuums into your plan then by the time your target weight has been reached your waistline will be all the more reduced.

4

Performing The Stomach Vacuum

Almost anybody can perform stomach vacuums and they can be done right away and with no previous experience or guidance. Stomach vacuums can be performed at any body fat level, by participants of any age, sex, or anything else. Unlike performing lifts such as the squat or clean and press, there's very little that can go wrong with a stomach vacuum and I've yet to hear of a single instance of an injury, a strain or anything else negative connected to them.

Part of the exercise is becoming more comfortable holding the position, as well as your breath, for ever longer periods of time. As with most things in life, this is something that will come with practice.

To execute the stomach vacuum:

1. Stand upright with your hands on hips (or assume one of the other positions below).
2. Prepare yourself for exhalation. I find that taking a

couple of deep, satisfying breaths can help.

3. Slowly exhale all the air from your lungs. At the same time slowly pull in your stomach. Ideally, you should reach full contraction of the TA muscle at the same time as you arrive at full expiration.

4. Once you feel the deepest part of your core engaged, you've got it! Hold this position.

5. A popular cue is to visualize trying to touch your navel to your backbone.

6. When you can no longer hold the contraction, release. That is one repetition.

7. Note the length of the repetition and write down if you're taking records.

8. Take a few moments to recover and repeat.

Tips

1. Executing stomach vacuums on a full stomach might feel uncomfortable when compared to performing them on an empty stomach. Likewise, doing the exercise with a full bladder might also impair performance. The best time to carry out stomach vacuums, therefore, might be first thing in the morning, after urination, when both your stomach and bladder are empty.

2. The limiting factor when it comes to your stomach vacuums will almost certainly be the amount of time you're able to hold the position without breathing. Although within time this will improve as you're able to hold your breath, and therefore the contraction, for ever longer periods of time, there's never any harm in taking small, sharp 'sips'

of breath in order to prolong the repetition. Whilst in the middle of a strong contraction, you will not feel your stomach expanding when taking one of these small breaths, and in doing so you can significantly draw out the length of the repetition.

3. For an extra variation, try thrusting out your ribcage, thus expanding your chest and creating a little more room in the target region. You'll almost certainly find the contraction will feel different, possibly even easier.

4. As with your usual exercise routine, try to get into a regular schedule of performing stomach vacuums. As with all things in life, the best results come from consistency.

5. Take measurements. Although recording waist circumference can conflate results if you're also dieting / training to lose body fat, by combining the tape measure with images taken in the mirror, you'll be doing as much as can reasonably be expected. We're unlikely to cut you open to measure the circumference of your TA because that would be wrong.

6. It shouldn't take long to master the basic technique, by which point the use of different positions should be encouraged.

Which brings us to the next section.

5

Positions

Once you've mastered the technique fundamentals you will almost certainly wish to experiment using different positions, which is the beauty of the stomach vacuum because it's something you can indeed do whilst lying back relaxing, waiting in line at the grocery store or even when you're stuck in traffic. Now you can turn what might otherwise have been wasted time into something productive.

In order of ascending difficulty, let's now take a look at a small number of useful positions.

Lying supine

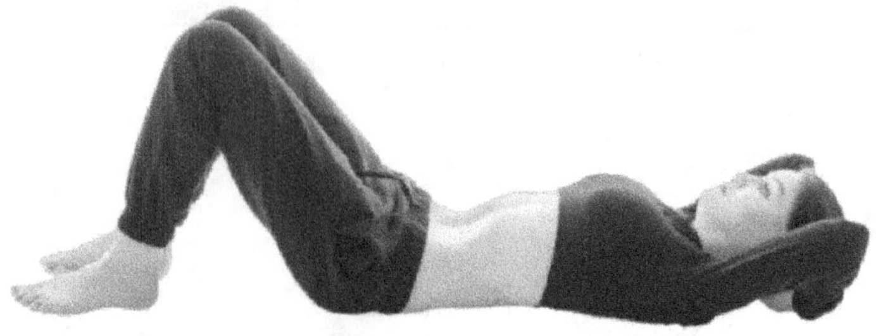

In the supine position you have an advantage because, thanks to gravity, lying down automatically draws in your stomach. If you perform your vacuums first thing in the morning with an empty stomach whilst still in bed then you might want to visualize pulling your abdomen into the mattress.

Bending at the waist

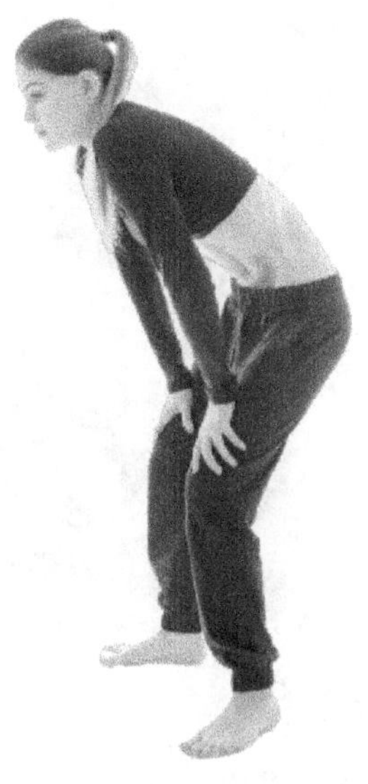

You might have noticed that bending forwards in such a way pushes out your belly. Performing stomach vacuums in this position, bending slightly forwards from the waist, compresses the stomach and allows for a deeper contraction of the diaphragm, and therefore the TA muscle, which will assist in the expulsion of more air from your lungs. This position allows for one of the best contractions performing the manoeuvre. You can complete the vacuum in this position or else stand once the air has been expelled, which again, owing to your abdomen being even more deeply pulled into your chest, should bring a different feeling.

Kneeling

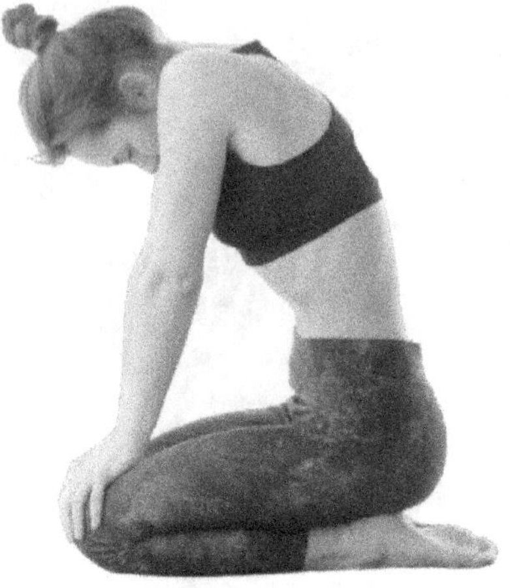

As with the above, this position compresses the stomach and diaphragm. The angle is closed even more and should therefore allow for an even greater contraction of the TA.

All-fours (quadruped position)

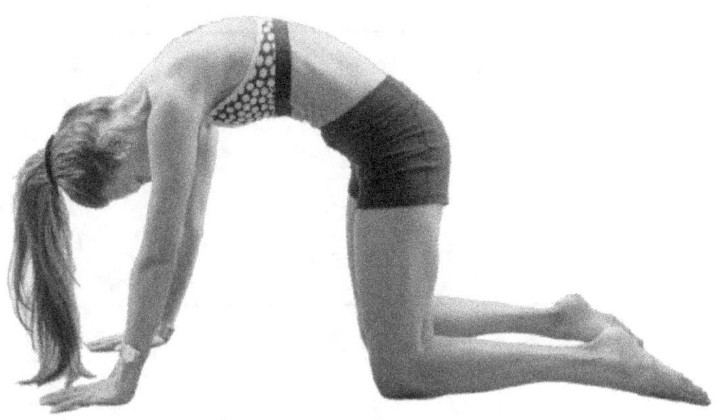

Of the four positions mentioned, one study [17] showed that the quadruped position is the most difficult to perform the vacuum. This is because you have to pull in your stomach against gravity.

6

Progression

Early results should be surprisingly visual and aesthetic, though as already stated, measurements of your waistline, as well as photographic images, should be taken so that you have physical evidence of the progress you're making.

As you become accustomed to and find performing stomach vacuums easier, then as with any training program, you'll want to gradually start ramping up the difficulty to ensure progress continues at a steady pace.

The variables you can change in order to progress are as follows:

- Repetitions
- Sets
- Duration of contraction
- Intensity
- Position

Repetitions & sets

When starting out you might be surprised by how much a single stomach vacuum takes out of you. As already stated, the TA muscle is one that's hardly ever contracted, certainly not with any form of deliberate targeting such as here, so at first you might only be able to perform one or two repetitions of the exercise.

One repetition refers to a single stomach vacuum, no matter how long it lasts or how intense the contraction. A set refers to how many repetitions are performed in a single exercise session. Sets can, and most likely will be, spread throughout the day.

$$Repetitions \; x \; Sets = Total$$

Over time you should aim to comfortably increase your total either by adding to the repetitions or sets, or a combination of both.

Duration

The amount of time you're able to hold a stomach vacuum will increase over time as you become more comfortable with the exercise. This, along with repetitions and sets, is something I would suggest keeping a record of, just so that you know you're making progress. Your first stomach vacuums could well last for as short a time as five seconds, though within a few weeks, you could well be reaching times as high as half a minute and beyond. Obviously, do not hold onto a contraction for so long that it becomes uncomfortable, and don't forget that you can take repeated 'sips' of air in order to draw it out. Don't forget that the stomach vacuum is an exercise for the transverse abdominis, breaking records for holding our breath is not the aim.

Intensity

As already mentioned, beginners might feel more comfortable not going all-out first time around. That's perfectly ok. In your head, rate the strength of your contractions on a scale of 1-10. You might want to start by contracting your TA muscle only to a five and then increase from there. However, let me be clear, because you will want to be reaching for those tens as soon as possible, as this is where the true power of the stomach vacuum is found.

How hard your TA is contracted will be one of the main determiners for how long you're able to hold it; the more purposefully you pull in, the shorter the duration is likely to be.

There will be times within a single repetition that you might unintentionally 'ease up,' not necessarily out of fatigue but because holding a stomach vacuum for any length of time actually requires a fair amount of concentration. A maximally contracted TA will yield the best results, irrespective of the duration of time you're able to hold it. If you engage in weightlifting then you might well have heard of the 'mind-muscle connection,' which perhaps can best be defined thus:

> "The mind-muscle connection is a conscious, deliberate, and emphasized muscle contraction. It requires focusing tension during a movement pattern specifically on the muscle or muscle group that should be working, and it makes all the difference between passively and actively moving the weight."

When performing your stomach vacuums, try placing all your concentration on the one muscle involved with the exercise and actually *feel* it with your mind as well as body. This should enable you to maintain a constant tension on the TA and make the most out of every contraction.

Position

Fairly self-explanatory. Try to get to the point where you're performing your stomach vacuums first thing in the morning, whilst lying face-up on the bed, either as you're sitting commuting or working at your desk, and then during the evening you could perhaps go for a more deliberate position on all-fours, which would mean a gradual increase in difficulty as the day progresses.

Anything else?

After you've mastered the stomach vacuum you might want to work on keeping your abdomen tight when you're sitting but also, especially, when you're out and about walking around throughout the day. By this, I don't mean an all-out full contraction but just enough so that your TA muscle remains active. Generally, this is good practice anyway, as walking with your stomach cinched in, your shoulders pulled back and your chin tilted up is good posture. Because your mind will then follow your body's cues, this will have the additional advantage of helping you to feel more confident, as well as appear taller.

Question: Can stomach vacuums be performed simultaneously with regular abdominal work?

It's definitely doable, and abdominal exercises are best performed with your stomach pulled in anyway, which will of course contract your TA muscle, however, whilst carrying out intense abdominal exercises breathing is hard enough as it is and in order to complete your sets satisfactorily then you'll want to maintain normal breathing rhythms. Those who've read my HIIT book will be aware that I'm not a fan of certain routines that combine two exercise modes, such as squatting or lunging whilst attempting the battle ropes, as I don't believe this to be the most efficient way of working maximally, at least not in the context of HIIT.

When it comes to stomach vacuums and ab crunches, do one or the other, separately if you must, for the best of all worlds.

7

Are There Any Potential Risks?

The truth is that I'm not sure I can think of a safer exercise to perform. In all my research I've not come across a single instance of anybody sustaining any injuries or accidents from performing a stomach vacuum.

However, there are a few instances where participants might wish to ease up on the intensity, before increasing the strength of their contractions from there, until they can be certain that performing stomach vacuums does not cause any pain or discomfort:

- If you are pregnant or suspect you might be pregnant.
- If you are in the middle of your menstrual period.
- If you suffer from an infectious disease in the stomach, such as colitis or gastritis.
- If you suffer from high blood pressure.

If any of these apply to you then again, start with an intensity of maybe 50%, along with a duration of just a few seconds, and gradually build up as per the progressions above.

8

Bonus Article

For purposes of completion, I'm including an article that covers all the bases and might hopefully benefit a great number of people reading these words.

Help! I'm Skinny But My Belly Sticks Out! What Can I Do To Fix It?

The majority of people reading this book will be most interested in reducing belly protrusion, flattening a convex appearance or even turning a flat belly into an inwardly curving concave shape. As we've learned, even if you possess a low level of body fat, it's still very possible for your belly to stick out. Irrespective of your present physical condition, if your belly protrudes it could be owing to one or more of several reasons which, you'll be pleased to know, stomach vacuums can attenuate more than one.

1. Your transverse abdominis muscle might be weak

I think I've already said it all with regards to this. The TA is a core muscle that holds in your internal organs. An underdeveloped TA could well result in your stomach sticking out and it matters not how long you can hold a plank, how many dragon flags you can perform or how shredded your six-pack might be because none of these things have much to do with the TA at all.

The fix: Strengthen your TA muscles to create a tighter coil around your internal organs.

2. Your posture might be poor

How you carry your own weight can have a dramatic effect not only on how others perceive you but also in how you perceive yourself. Ever notice how much more confident you feel when you walk with your shoulders pulled back and your chin tilted up? It's a matter of your mind following the cues from your body which, in turn, will then have a positive effect back on your mind.

The midsection is an important part of your overall posture. If your posture is poor then it will likely manifest, at least to some extent, with a protruding belly.

In the short term, the fix is to practice good postural habits. Starting from the base and working up, I like to walk with my hips thrust forwards just a touch more than what might feel normal. By doing this there's less effort required up top. As already discussed, one should habitually pull in their stomach. It's the shoulders, however, which are a problem for a great many people, as modern living often necessitates a weak back which results in the shoulders rounding forwards over time. As stated, pulling back the shoulders whilst consciously tilting up the chin will be far less effort if you're pushing out just a touch from the hips, as this will alter the angle of your torso.

Over the long term, it's important to incorporate good habits into your lifestyle. Stomach vacuums will strengthen the TA, which within time will improve posture without having to consciously think about it. Additionally, strength training can have all kinds of miraculous effects on your wellbeing, poor posture being just one of the things that can be attenuated by use of a range of back exercises in particular, the most important being the face pull, which targets the muscles that counter those in the chest that pull on and round the shoulders forwards.

The fix: Practice good postural techniques, stomach vacuums and strength training exercises.

3. You might have lordosis

A small amount of inward curvature of the spine's lumbar region is completely normal, however, when the curve becomes too excessive then it's defined as lordosis, and it's not hard to understand why such a condition would cause your stomach to stick out.

Lordosis is usually caused by an imbalance of musculature surrounding the pelvis, a combination of weak abdominal muscles and hip flexors, and tight back extensors.

Unfortunately, this seems to be another consequence of modernity, sitting and slouching for long hours at desks.

Difficulty moving, lower back pain and muscle spasms might be signs you have lordosis, at least to some degree. To know for sure then lie back on the ground and place your hand beneath the curvature of your lower back. If the gap is excessive, if you're able to move your hand around freely, then this could be an indicator.

Again, this is something that good habits can cure. Strengthening the muscles of the abdomen, this time with planks, crunches and leg raises along with, you guessed it, stomach vacuums, will go a long way to making improvements. A full-body strength training program, once again, will give the surrounding musculature a good balance. In addition, one should carry out more stretching, particularly in the muscles that are known to become tight such as the hamstrings.

The fix: Strength training, particularly abdominal exercises including stomach vacuums, and stretches.

4. You might be skinny-fat

Being skinny-fat, the most notable manifestation will be a loss of muscle mass, making one appear lean in the chest, arm, shoulder and even leg region, and an increase in fat mass, most prominently in the stomach, for men, or the thighs and buttocks for women.

Yet another consequence of modernity; long hours in seated positions and lifestyles that require little to no physical exertion whilst maintaining the same caloric input might well, over the months and years, result in becoming skinny-fat. Conversely, however, a badly thought through training program, one that contains an excessive amount of steady-state cardio coupled with a low-calorie intake, perhaps in a concerted effort at combatting the skinny-fat look, might well result in maintaining this condition or even making it worse. High estrogen along with low testosterone levels are little help either.

Thankfully, the fix is very doable and even enjoyable. It should come as no real surprise that strength training will increase muscle mass, which in turn will increase your metabolic rate and fat burning potential. Cleaning up your diet; cutting out sugar and increasing the quantity of lean proteins is essential. Finally, ditch the steady-state cardio for HIIT, a training regimen that's been found [16] to be nine times more efficient at burning fat whilst taking up less than half the time. Doing just those things alone will take care of any hormonal imbalances (estrogen/testosterone) that you might have.

The fix: Strength training, HIIT and an improved diet.

5. Menopause could be to blame

Women usually store fat in the thighs, hips and buttocks, but after menopause their body shape typically changes. With the onset of menopause there's a decrease in levels of estrogen and this, in turn, causes more fat to store around the belly.

The good news is that when it comes to post-menopausal belly fat, there's no secret when it comes to losing it. A reduction in processed foods and sugars, along with an increase in healthy fats and proteins is suggested. Other than that, strength training is always a wonderful idea, as is engaging in regular HIIT workouts.

The fix: Good diet, strength training, HIIT workouts.

6. Stress

Although small amounts of stress can be a great motivator and can literally haul your arse out of bed to start doing things, too much of it can have some serious problems. A lack of energy, headaches, nausea, stomach aches, bodily aches and pains, a rapid heartbeat, insomnia, frequent colds, loss of libido, becoming easily agitated and moody, depression, worrying, forgetfulness, an inability to focus, poor judgement, pessimism, procrastination, exhibiting more nervous behaviours such as nail-biting and fidgeting, a loss or problematic gain in appetite and an increased use of drugs, alcohol and cigarettes are just some of the short term symptoms. Longer term we can add an even greater number of mental health problems, cardiovascular disease, heart disease, high blood pressure, heart attacks, stroke, menstrual problems, sexual dysfunction such as impotence, skin and hair problems such as acne, psoriasis, eczema and permanent hair loss, obesity and eating disorders to this awful list of woes.

Cortisol is made in the adrenal gland and is known as the body's stress hormone. It's elevated when we experience stress or anxiety, and is lowered when we relax. Cortisol is essential for survival, it increases glucose in the bloodstream and helps to repair tissues, but too much of it is another symptom of stress - and the thing about cortisol is that too much of it forces the body to store any excess calories, which by the way you're possibly intaking as a symptom of stress, in the belly instead of all over the body.

An excess of stress really is one of those things you must keep out of your life, for all sorts of reasons. Manage your stress by exercising regularly, strength training and, yet again, HIIT, taking leisurely walks preferably out in nature, meditating, and if it can be helped, by not placing yourself in stressful situations to begin with.

The fix: Strength training, HIIT, walking, meditation, destressing your life.

7. Genetics

It won't surprise anybody to learn that genetics plays a major role in the shape of our bodies, including where fat is stored and in what quantities. Your assigned-at-birth somatotype determines the shape of your body with endomorphs, those with short limbs in comparison to their torso, being more likely to store fat around the midsection.

Since there's nothing you can do to change your somatotype, you're left with two options; either give up because you were dealt a bad hand or make the most of the cards you were given.

Never allow genetics to be an easy let-off for not taking action. Even if nature does indeed supersede nurture (and I'm not getting into that debate here), and even if that question was heavily lopsided in favour of genetics, that small amount of nurture, something which you certainly are in control of, can still move mountains. As being born poor or in the wrong neighbourhood is an easy way to excuse one's lot in life, using such an excuse as genetics is likewise a convenient way to rob ourselves of agency over our own destinies.

The fix: Train, eat, sleep, repeat.

8. Smoking

Nicotine is known to suppress appetite, which in turn promotes an unhealthy way of losing weight. However, one study [19] found that "for a given BMI, increased cigarette consumption was associated with an increased waist circumference. Smoking in an effort to control weight may lead to accumulation of central adiposity." In other words, smoking reduces overall weight but actually increases waist circumference.

By now, I shouldn't have to tell anybody that quitting smoking is the single most advantageous health improving measure one can ever take, and is in fact the only thing that beats out even strength training.

The fix: Quit smoking.

Message From The Author

Thank you so much for making it this far.

Can a few minutes a day performing this strange exercise really constrict your waistline and reduce the size of your stomach? Absolutely! But if you need any further convincing then I would urge you to peruse some of the anecdotes that you'll find around the web from some of the many people who've had great success with the stomach vacuum.

But if you're still sceptical then I would encourage you to give it your best efforts for just one month to see what results you might have. If nothing happens then you've lost nothing.

Fair?

If, on the other hand, you're fully convinced then now all you need to do is take action and commit to a regular schedule, in which case, again, just give yourself a month to see what happens.

Good luck with it!

If you've enjoyed this book and feel that others might also benefit from the material contained within then please don't hesitate to leave an honest review on the page where you made the purchase. It really does make all the difference. Alternatively, you can simply leave a quick rating on your device.

Thanks and best wishes.

James Driver

Also by James Driver

HIIT: High Intensity Interval Training Explained

Tired of Feeling Tired: Destroy Fatigue and Re-Energize your Life.

References

1. Lum et al (2019). Brief Review: Effects of Isometric Strength Training on Strength and Dynamic Performance.

https://pubmed.ncbi.nlm.nih.gov/30943568/

2. Lum et al (2021). Sprint Kayaking Performance Enhancement by Isometric Strength Training Inclusion: A Randomized Controlled Trial.

https://pubmed.ncbi.nlm.nih.gov/33494230/

3. Lee et al (2018). Do isometric, isotonic and/or isokinetic strength trainings produce different strength outcomes?

https://pubmed.ncbi.nlm.nih.gov/29861246/

4. Oranchuk et al (2018). Isometric training and long-term adaptations: Effects of muscle length, intensity, and intent: A systematic review.

https://onlinelibrary.wiley.com/doi/10.1111/sms.13375

5. Willett et al (2001). Relative activity of abdominal muscles during commonly prescribed strengthening exercises.

https://pubmed.ncbi.nlm.nih.gov/11726260/

6. Casonatto et al (2019). Pilates exercise and postural balance in older adults: A systematic review and meta-analysis of randomized controlled trials.

https://pubmed.ncbi.nlm.nih.gov/31987246/

7. Watson et al (2017). Dance, Balance & Core Muscle Performance Measures Are Improved Following A 9-Week Core Stabilization Training Program Among Competitive Collegiate Dancers.

https://pubmed.ncbi.nlm.nih.gov/28217414/

8. Moreno-Muñoz (2021). The Effects of Abdominal Hypopressive Training on Postural Control and Deep Trunk Muscle Activation: A Randomized Controlled Trial. International Journal of Environmental Research and Public Health 18(5):2741

9. Oh et al (2020). Comparison of Effects of Abdominal Draw-In Lumbar Stabilization Exercises with and without Respiratory Resistance on Women with Low Back Pain: A Randomized Controlled Trial.

https://pubmed.ncbi.nlm.nih.gov/32182226/

10. Sprestad et al (2016). Diastasis recti abdominis during pregnancy and 12 months after childbirth: prevalence, risk factors and report of lumbopelvic pain.

https://www.ncbi.nlm.nih.gov/pmc/
articles/PMC5013086/

11. Chiarello et al (2005). The effects of an exercise program on diastasis recti abdominis in pregnant women. J Womens Health Phys Ther;29(1):11–16.

12. Laframboise et al (2021). Postpartum Exercise Intervention Targeting Diastasis Recti Abdominis.

https://www.ncbi.nlm.nih.gov/pmc/
articles/PMC8136546/

13. Litos (2014). Progressive therapeutic exercise program for successful treatment of a postpartum woman with a severe diastasis recti abdominis. J Womens Health Phys Ther. 2014;38(2):58–73.

14. Benjamin et al (2014). Effects of exercise on diastasis of the rectus abdominis muscle in the antenatal and postnatal periods: a systematic review.

https://pubmed.ncbi.nlm.nih.gov/24268942/

15. Álvarez Sáez et al (2016). Can an eight-week program based on the hypopressive technique produce changes in pelvic floorfunction and body composition in female rugby players?

https://core.ac.uk/reader/32326819

16. Tremblay A, et al. (1994). Impact of Exercise Intensity on Body Fatness and Skeletal Muscle Metabolism. *Metabolism: Clinical and Experimental*. 43(7):814-8.

http://www.ncbi.nlm.nih.gov/pubmed/8028502

17. Moghadam et al (2019). Comparison of the recruitment of transverse abdominis through drawing-in and bracing in different core stability training positions.

https://pubmed.ncbi.nlm.nih.gov/31938704

18. Dallman et al (2004). Minireview: glucocorticoids--food intake, abdominal obesity, and wealthy nations in 2004.

https://pubmed.ncbi.nlm.nih.gov/15044359/

19. Morris et al (2015). Heavier smoking may lead to a relative increase in waist circumference: evidence for a causal relationship from a Mendelian randomisation meta-analysis. The CARTA consortium.

https://www.ncbi.nlm.nih.gov/pmc/
articles/PMC4538266/

www.ingramcontent.com/pod-product-compliance
Lightning Source LLC
Chambersburg PA
CBHW060913130726

48001CB00006B/2212